THIS BOOK BELONGS TO

The Library of

....

....

Thank you for Purchasing my book and taking the time to read it from front to back. I am always grateful when a reader chooses my work and I hope you enjoyed it!

With the vast selection available online, I am touched that you chose to be purchasing my work and take valuable time out of your life to read it. My hope is that you feel you made the right decision.

I very much would like to know what you thought of the book. Please take the time to write an honest and informative review on Amazon.com. Your experience and opinions will be of great benefit to me and those readers looking to make an informed choice.

With much thanks.

Table of Contents

Introduction

I would like to thank you for downloading this book,

This book contains proven steps and strategies on how to burn body fat, lose weight and eat healthy.

Are you on the verge of giving up on your weight loss goals? Have you tried reducing your fat intake, eating fewer carbohydrates and all the diets that call for eating fewer proteins and carbohydrates, drank a lot of water, but you don't lose any weight? Does nothing seem to work?Well, I guess losing hope is understandable, but wait, DO NOT GIVE UP JUST YET! There is one more option, the best option in fact.

If we are to go by the facts, theNegative Calorie Diet is the fastest way to lose weight; you can lose up to 14 pounds a week when you adopt the diet! Thanks to this diet, losing weight is no longer a random dream or a hope; it is a reality for thousands of people across the globe.

In this book, you will learn more about the Negative Calorie Diet, how it works and some amazing recipes that will help you burn fat.

Thanks again for downloading this book, I hope you enjoy it!

Negative Calorie Diet: What Is It

This unique diet draws upon theidea that some foodshave the 'negative caloric' effect that we ought to consider in burning fat. A food is considered to have a negative calorie effect when the calories these foods use to digest are typically higherthan the calories in the foods themselves.

When you eat something, you begin by chewing, a process that consumes energy. Some foods such as those higher in stringy fibers like celery will require more chewing, which will result in more energy expenditure, and there are otherslike pasta and cakes that don't require as much chewing.

After chewing, the foods go to the stomach through the esophagus and the other processes of digestion take over until absorption takes place and the body excretes the residual mass.

With negative calorie foods, this entire process uses up more calories than the foods have. The extra calories the body has to provide in order to process the foods are taken from the fat stores, and the more of these negative calorie foods you eat, the more your fat stores will lose calories, and as a result, the more fatyou will lose.

Let us take broccoli as an example: 100 grams (contains 25 calories).

When you eat 100 grams of broccoli, it takes your body about 80 calories worth of energy to digest it. This results in a net calorie use of 55 calories that should come from the fat stores in your body. As you can see, the 55 calories make up the negative net calorie.

Let us now take a counter example of a piece of cake containing 400 calories.

Your body will take about 150 calories to digest the piece of cake, leaving net 250 caloriesdeposited in the body and stored as fat.

The negative calorie diet consists of over 100 foods proven to have negative calorie qualities. Most of these foods are fruits and veggies that are high in fiber. Let us look at them in more detail in the following chapter.

Negative Calorie Food List

Here is a list of negative calorie foods:

Vegetables

Vegetables are highly nutritious and not high in calories when compared to many processed foods. Nonetheless, some vegetables are superior especially when it comes to the negative calorie food list. The following are vegetables you should consider including in your diet.

Artichokes	Bean sprouts	Broccoli	Cabbage	Cauliflower
Asparagus	Beets and beet greens	Brussels sprouts	Carrots	Celery
Chives	Cucumbers	Green beans	Mushrooms	Peppers (red, green, yellow)
Pumpkin	Sauerkraut	Spinach	String beans	Turnips
Corn	Eggplant	Lettuce	Peas	Pickles
Radishes	Scallions	Squash	Tomatoes	Zucchini
Garlic	Onion	Watercress		

Fruits

Just like vegetables, fruits are a healthier option and always the recommended healthy alternative to sugary foods. It is therefore a better idea to snack on a bunch of grapes than it is to snack on candy.

However, when it comes to fruit choices, you also need to make better choices because some fruits are high in calories; thus, not providing you the negative calorie effect you are looking for in negative calorie foods

The list below contains some good negative-calorie fruits you can eat:

Apples	Blackberries	Cantaloupe	Cranberries	Grapefruit
Honeydew melon	Lemons	Mangoes	Apricots	Blueberries

Cherries	Currants	Grapes	Kiwi	Limes
Nectarines	Oranges	Pears	Pomegranates	Strawberries
Watermelon	Peaches	Pineapple	Raspberries	Tangerines
Prunes				

It is important to remember that while some fruits and vegetables are negative calorie foods, this does not mean that you can go ahead and consume them in juice form. As we've seen, a lot of energy is expended when chewing food. Juicing means that you skip this important action. Thus, your body will not burn as much energy as it would have if you were to chew the foods.

Herbs and spices

When it is a question of what you eat, even herbs and spices matter. Below is a complete list of herbs and spices you should always go for.

Chili pepper	Cloves	Ginger	Parsley	Cinnamon
Mustard seeds	Cayenne	Anise	Coriander/Cilantro	Dill
Cumin	Fennel seeds			

The good thing about herbs and spices is that they can be sprinkled in a variety of dishes. You can use them to add flavor to cooked food. You can also add them to soup and gravy. In addition, you can definitely use them in salads. Thus, go ahead and find opportunities to use these useful negative calorie foods.

Meat, Fish and Seafood

Red meat can be harmful to you, and many negative calorie diets don't recommend it; however, you do not have to avoid eating meat altogether, as it provides essential proteins and other nutrients. A good source of protein is fish for instance. Fish is lower in calories but high in essential nutrients like omega-3 fatty acids.

If you are allergic to fish, or if you are not a big fan of it, you can alternatively include small/reasonable potions of meat and chicken in your diet (I will teach you how in the recipes section).

The table below shows some of the best fish and seafood to include in your diet:

Clams	Crayfish	Mussels	Shrimp	Crab
Flounder	Tuna	Abalone	Buffalo fish	Cod
Terrapin	Bass	Catfish	Trout	

How To Make The Transition To Negative Calorie Diet

Now that you know what to eat, let us see exactly how you are going to be eating all that.

1. Make a smooth transition into the negative calorie diet so that you are comfortable with the entire process. Start by adding some negative calorie foods to the foods you normally eat in every meal in the 1:1 ratio. For instance, if having pasta with meatballs, you can serve 50% of this food and add chunks of zucchini to fill the other half.

You can also add a mixed salad to each meal you have; the salad should comprise of not less than 90% negative calorie foods. This means you have to look for ways to substitute any unwanted content such as any creamy high-fat substances with something like raspberry vinaigrette.

After some time, start slowly substituting the foods with the good (negative calorie) ones until your plate contains up to 90% negative calorie foods.

Note: We are only adding vegetables and fruits so far, not necessarily fully prepared negative calorie meals. Next, we will discuss the recipes so that you have entirely cooked meals too.

2.Use several vegetables to make a stir-fry. You can also make smoothie shakes with your favorite fruits including some berries. As said before, the negative calorie diet is largely a fruits and vegetables diet. However, this does not mean you should now start worrying about how you will survive as a vegetarian.

You can occasionallyenjoy small servings of chicken and some meat, and the recipes in the following chapter will reflect that. Nonetheless, the meats have to be in small amounts; remember, you are losing weight and so, you have to make some sacrifices.

First Thing to Do

Buy all the foods you think you require from the list, wash, cut them into bits thon coal them in airtight containers for storage (in the fridge) so that you will have them handy anytime you need them. You do not want to come home from work tired in the evening without having a bunch of these foods readily available. If you do, you will be extremely tempted to grab something unhealthy.

If you are wondering whether you will be hungry on this diet plan, just know that you will not because these foods are filling because they are high in fiber as well as water; the perfect combination to be full.

Note: While on this diet, you should have no room for alcohol, sugar, or any sugar substitutes except stevia simply because sugar intake causes your body to produce more insulin. This hormone signals/tells the fat cells to pick up and convert any excess glucose into fat. Therefore, eating more sugar means more production of insulin and consequently, more deposits in the fat cells. We are trying to reduce fat in your body, not create more of it. In this regard, avoid all commercial dressings since most of them contain sugar and high fat content.

Now that we have that out of the way, let us start cooking!

Negative Calorie Diet Recipes

While on a strict diet (such as this one), you might have a problem trying to decide what kind of dressing to use for your meals. Since I know it is important to be careful about what you are using, I will start by giving you two simple dressings that you will use on any meal you want.

Garlic and Herbs Dressing

Mix 1/2 cup of cold-pressed extra-virgin olive oil with juice from 1 lemon, 2 crushed garlic cloves and ¼ cup apple cider vinegar. Add some of your favorite negative caloriedried herbs such as parsley and cilantro.

This will yield 1 cup of dressing. Store the dressing in the fridge (for up to one month) to use on your foods.

Dijon and Yoghurt Dressing

For a delicious vegetable dip, mix Dijon mustard (2 tablespoons) with 2 cups low-fat yoghurt then add a pinch of chili pepper and a teaspoon of mixed dried herbs to spice it up.

Breakfast Recipes

Pumpkin Pancakes

Serves 4

Ingredients

1 cup of canned pumpkin

1 1/4 cups of water

2 teaspoons of cinnamon

2 cups Krusteaz pancake mix

1 egg, slightly beaten

1 teaspoon of baking powder

For the topping

1/4 cup of sliced pecans

5 tablespoons of pure maple syrup

Instructions

Combine all the ingredients for the pancake batter.

On a griddle or pan over medium heat sprayed with a little cooking spray, create a 10 cm circle of batter.

When the pancakes turn brown at the edges and you notice even bubbling across the top, flip them over to cook the other side.

In the meantime, toast pecans in a small pan until they turn slightly brown and give out the fragrance.

Serve with heated pure maple syrup.

Apple and Cinnamon with Almonds and Oat Bran

Serves 4

Ingredients

4 large apples

1 teaspoon of ground cinnamon

1/4 cup of oat bran

10 almonds, toasted and chopped

1 teaspoon of unrefined coconut oil

2 cups of unsweetened vanilla almond milk

2 packets monk fruit extract

Instructions

Wash the apples and cut into cubes.

Melt the coconut oil in a large nonstick skillet over medium high heat. Add the cinnamon and apples then cook for 2-3 minutes until the apples soften.

Remove from the heat, add almond milk, stir in the monk fruit extract and oat bran. Once mixed return back to the heat, stir, and bring to a simmer.

Cook for about one minute, until the mixture becomes thick and creamy.

Divide the mixture among four bowls then sprinkle each one with toasted almonds.

Negative Calorie Smoothie

Serves 2

Ingredients

5 strawberries

½ medium papaya

1 grapefruit

¼ cup ice

Instructions

Put all the ingredients in a blender; blend until smooth.

Serve and garnish with some strawberries and enjoy.

Lunch Recipes

Vegetable Soup

Serves 6

This is not your regular veggie soup; yes, it is simple, but it is full of negative calorie foods only.

Ingredients

6 cups of vegetable stock

1 cup of celery, diced

1 cup of green beans cut into about 1 inch pieces

1 medium zucchini, diced (approximately 2 cups)

1 cup small turnip, diced

1 jalapeno, seeded and finely chopped

1 medium onion, diced

1 cup of cauliflower florets

2 cups of shredded cabbage

3 cloves of garlic, finely chopped

2 cups of baby spinach

Salt and pepper to taste

Instructions

Mix the ingredients (except the spinach) in a pot, and bring to a boil.

Cover and let it simmer for 20 minutes.

Add the spinach, stir, and let it cook for one more minute.

Remove from the heat and serve.

Toast with Tomatoes

Serves 4

Ingredients

8 cups of spinach

½ ripe avocado, mashed well with a fork

Salt to taste

Freshly ground black pepper to taste

4 slices of natural gluten-free bread

4 (½-inch) slices ripe tomato

4 eggs, poached

Green hot sauce

Instructions

Place a nonstick skillet over medium high heat.

Add the spinach and cook until it wilts. Move the spinach to a colander and strain out as much water as possible. Put the now drained spinach in a bowl and season with green hot sauce and salt.

Use a toaster to toast the bread then season the avocado with salt. Evenly spreadthe pieces of avocado over each piece of toast then add a slice of tomato on top. Use pepper and salt to season the tomatoes and use the spinach mixture to top each slice evenly.

Place every piece of toast on a fresh plate. Finally, top with a poached egg and serve.

Meatballs with Mushroom Gravy

Serves 4

Ingredients

12 ounces lean ground beef

1 ounce Parmigiano Reggiano cheese, finely chopped

2 tablespoons arrowroot, dissolved in 2 teaspoons of stock

8 cups washed spinach

1 cup thinly sliced onion

4 cups sliced cremini mushrooms

Olive oil cooking spray

Freshly ground black pepper

Salt to taste

4 cups unsalted beef stock

1 cup finely chopped puffed brown rice

Instructions

Put the beef in a large bowl and push it to one side. Add rice and a cup of the stock to the other side of the mixing bowl; season with pepper and salt and allow the rice to absorb the stock for about 1 minute.

Mix the beef and rice using an electric hand mixture until well mixed. Taste and adjust the seasoning then use the mixture to form 16 meatballs.

Coat a skillet with olive oil cooking spray and place over medium heat. Once hot, put the meatballs and brown for one minute on one side. Turn and brown the opposite side for around 30 seconds and transfer to a plate.

Add the mushrooms to the skillet and sauté for a few minutes. Add the meatballs back to the skillet, then add the beef stock, arrowroot mixture, and cook until meatballs are cooked through.

Add the spinach and season with pepper and salt and cook until the spinach is wilted. Add the cheese, stir, and serve.

Dinner Recipes

Brussels Sprouts with Lemon and Almond Dressing

Serves 3-4

Ingredients

3 pints Brussels sprouts, shaved thinly

5 teaspoons of freshly minced garlic

Crushed red pepper flakes

1/2 cup of chopped fresh flat-leaf parsley

Salt

1 1/2 teaspoons of extra-virgin olive oil

1/4 cup of toasted almonds, finely chopped

1/8 teaspoon of ground cinnamon

1/2 cup freshly squeezed lemon juice

1 ounce of Parmigiano-Reggiano cheese, finely grated

Instructions

Place the Brussels in a large mixing bowl and place it aside.

Placea non-stick skillet over medium high heat then add the garlic and olive oil. Cook until the garlic turns deep golden brown. Remove from the heat then add the parsley, almonds, cinnamon, and red pepper flakes.

Return the skillet back to the heat sauté for about ten seconds.Remove from the heat, pour in the lemon juice, and then season with salt.

Add the dressing to the Brussels then toss well, add 75% of the cheese, and toss some more. Taste then add the seasoning and top with the rest of the cheese.

Chicken with Pesto

Serves 3 or 4

Ingredients

Water

6 garlic cloves, chopped

Dash of paprika

1 cup of fresh basil leaves

8 cups ofchopped escarole

Salt

1 ounce of Parmigiano-Reggiano cheese, finely grated

Olive oil cooking spray

Dash of cinnamon

Crushed red pepper flakes

1 small onion, thinly sliced

4 cups chicken stock,unsalted

12 ounces of skinless, boneless chicken breast sliced into 1/8 inch thick strips

Instructions

Pour 2 quarts of water in a medium pot and bring to a simmer. You will use this to poach the chicken.

Lightly coat a medium skillet with olive oil cooking spray then place it over medium high heat.

Add the garlic and cook until it turns golden brown. Add the cinnamon, basil leaves, red pepper flakes, onion, and paprika. Cook for roughly 2 minutes until the onion softens.

Add the escarole then cook until it is soft and wilted – for 2 more minutes. Add the stock, bring to a simmer, and then cover. Cook for about 5 minutes or until tender.

Add a pinch of salt to the simmering water and turn off the heat. Add the chicken and stir well until all parts separate. Cook until you notice the strips turning white (meaning they are half cooked). Use a slotted spoon to transfer the strips to a plate to cool.

Let the remaining mixture cook until most of the stock evaporates and looks like thick sauce or soup. Turn off the heat.

Add in half of the cheese, stir, and then season with salt to taste. Add the chicken strips then toss them to coat with the mixture and keep cooking until the strips have cooked enough through, for about 90 seconds.

Top with the remaining cheese, and then serve.

Vegetable Beef Soup

Serves 14

Note: This recipe has many ingredients and it is likely you will hate some vegetables or herbs. You can replace these vegetables and herbs with other ingredients on the negative calorie food list.

Ingredients

4 chopped onions

1 chopped red bell pepper

4 cups of sliced fresh mushrooms

10 chopped celery stalks with their leaves

2 cupsof fresh chopped broccoli

1 small chopped bunch of cilantro

5 box low sodium beef broth

1 large chopped green bell pepper

4 cups of chopped cabbage

6 large chopped fresh carrots

1 finely chopped head of garlic

6 cups of fresh chopped spinach

1 small bunch of Parsley

1 canof asparagus (drained)

2 cans of green beans (drained)

1 cupof canned artichokes (drained)

20 twists of cracked black pepper

1 tablespoon of Italian seasoning

Protein (you can use just about any meat preferably the <u>fishes mentioned in the list</u>)

2 10 oz. cans of tomatoes with green chili's (not drained)

2 cans of diced tomatoes with basil (not drained)

1/2 tablespoon of red pepper flakes

1 tablespoonof dried basil

2 small cans of chopped green chilies (not drained)

1 lb. 80/20 or leaner ground beef (drain if needed)

Instructions

Fill a large cooking pot halfway with the beef, chicken, or vegetable stock. Add all the canned ingredients while draining some as specified intothe pot.

Add water and all the spices then stir. Let it boil for some time, lower the heat to simmer for one hour or until the vegetables soften.

As the soup boils down, add some extra broth and stir.

Serve, garnish as desired, and enjoy.

Snacks

Apple Chips

Serves 2

Ingredients

2 large granny smith apples

1 teaspoon of stevia

1 teaspoon of cinnamon

Canola oil cooking spray

Instructions

Preheat your oven to 200 degrees.

Using a sharp knife, thinlyslice the apples crosswise. Arrange the slices on a single layer on a baking sheet then spray with canola oil cooking spray.

Evenlysprinkle the stevia and cinnamon over the apple slices.

Use the bottom third part of the oven to bake the apples until they are crisp and dry, roughly 2-2½ hours.

Alternatively, you could use a mastrad chipmaker. Not only is it easy and fast, you do not need the cooking spray. Just lay the apple slices on the chipmaker, sprinkle with cinnamon and stevia, and then microwave for 4-5 minutes.

Berry Salad

Serves 4

Ingredients

4 cups of mixed berries (blackberries, raspberries, blueberries, strawberries)

20 whole almonds, toasted and chopped

2 tablespoons of hemp hearts

1/4 cup of cooked quinoa

1 ½ tablespoons of fat free yoghurt

Instructions

Equally divide all the ingredients among four bowls and toss well to mix.

Fruit Salad

Serves 10

Ingredients

2/3 cup of fresh orange juice

1/2 teaspoon of grated lemon zest

2 cups of cubed fresh pineapple

3 kiwi fruits, peeled and sliced

2 oranges, peeled and sectioned

2 cups of blueberries

1/3 cup of fresh lemon juice

1/2 teaspoon of grated orange zest

1 teaspoon of vanilla extract

2 cups of strawberries, hulled and sliced

3 bananas, sliced

1 cup seedless grapes

Instructions

Add orange zest, orange juice, lemon juice and lemon zest, to a saucepan, place it over medium high heat, and bring to boil.

Decrease the heat to medium-low and let it simmer for 5 minutes. Remove from the heat and stir in the vanilla extract. Place it aside to cool.

Place the fruit in a clear glass bowl in layers starting with the pineapple, then strawberries, kiwi, bananas, oranges, then grapes and at the top, blueberries.

Pour the juice over the fruit layers then cover and leave in the fridge for 3-4 hours before serving.

Almond Cake with Berries

Serves 4

Ingredients

½ cup of almond meal

4 packets of monk fruit extract

1 teaspoon of vanilla extract

Olive oil cooking spray

2 eggs, separated; remove 1 yolk

3 tablespoons of raw coconut nectar

Salt

1 cup of mixed berries, mashed well with a fork

Instructions

Preheat your oven to 3750 degrees F.

Bake the almond meal until it becomes aromatic and well toasted – about 3-5 minutes. Remove from the oven and place it on a cool baking sheet.

Place the monk fruit and egg whites in a bowl and whisk until it forms stiff peaks. Use cooking spray to spray four paper cups. Using a toothpick or fork, poke holes in the bottom of each.

Place the almond meal into a mixing bowl then add the egg yolk, salt, vanilla, and coconut nectar. Fold the meringue into the mixture of almond and transfer the batter into the cups.

Place in the microwave and microwave for about thirty seconds. When the mixture has cooked through, place the cups on their sides and give them 45 seconds to cook.

Remove the cakes and place themupside down on four serving plates.

Get them off the cups and serve with berries.

Cucumber and salsa

Serves 2

Ingredients

2 cucumbers, peeled and sliced

12 garlic cloves, minced

¼ cup fresh cilantro, chopped

3 tomatoes, diced

½ sweet onion, diced

Sea salt and black pepper to taste

Instructions

Mix all ingredients except the cucumber in a bowl in order to make the salsa.

Place cucumber slices on a plate and serve with the salsa.

Negative Calorie Diet And Exercise: An Effective Way To Lose Weight Fast

I promised you some unique and cool exercise tips, right? Doing the following exercises will help you burn the fat much faster. All you have to do is to start slow and over time, increase the intensity, keep an open mind, and use the gym (for the ones that require it), where you have an instructor nearby.

Interval Training

This is all about high intensity exercises combined with short periods of rest. This will not only burn more calories than your typical cardio training, it will boost your body's ability to burn fat easily since it increases the production of the growth hormone, which is also a fat burning hormone, and adrenaline which assists in suppressing your appetite.

The intervals will work on your muscles, and help them use oxygen better so that your heart does not have to struggle to pump a lot to make them perform.

Do It!

Get on a treadmill or a stationary bike then use the guide below to start your own interval-training regimen:

Begin with a regular warm-up (any simple exercise to get your blood rushing). When done, run or pedal at a rate that is more than your regular cardio intensity by 20%. If you have never engaged in any serious cardio workouts before, you might want to check this first to understand what I am talking about.

After 30 seconds to 1 minute, reduce the intensity to a rate that is 50% less than the intensity of a regular cardio workout. Alternate the periods of 30 seconds to 1 minute of hard work with 30 seconds to 1 minute of relaxed pedaling or if you want, relaxed running for 6-10 intervals to finish your session.

As this gets simpler, increase each interval's intensity so that you work even longer during the difficult part, reduce your rest periods, or if you feel enthusiastic enough, add more intervals.

Repeat 3-4 times each week.

As you get the hang of this exercise, start the next:

Sprinting

Try sprinting up a hill since the impact on your joints will be much lower and can help you avoid injury. If there is no hilly ground in your area, try the alternative: the dag race approach. Start your sprint by increasing your speed from a jog.

To make the most of this exercise, keep the sprints short – ideally50 yards per sprint. This helps you sustain a high intensity all through and prevents injury.

If you want to increase the overall results of your sprint workout, increase your total number of sprints. This is better than going for long distance runs.

If you are new to exercising, do not do more than one workout per week. You can increase the days once you accustom to the exercise; just remember to allow at least two days of recovery between the workouts.

As you get the hang of the above exercise, start the next:

High Intensity Strength Intervals

Select two exercises that work different muscles completely or ones that use opposite movements. For instance, you can pair a pulling exercise with a pushing exercise or upper body exercise with a lower body exercise like pull-ups and squats.

For the latter, select a weight (if your instructor thinks you need one) with which you can do 10 repetitions. Alternate between the two exercises and do just five repetitions of each move in every set. Remember to rest between the sets so that you finish each set without failing.

Keep alternating between the exercises for a 10 or 15 minutes set time. Keep noting the total number of sets you can do. In subsequent sessions, try to beat your score by completing more sets in the same duration or completing the same number of sets but with heavier weights.

As you get the hang of the above exercises, start the next:

Countdown Workouts

Countdown workouts fit in the use of exercise pairs really well. They also keep you fully engaged in the exercises since you have to keep the count and pay attention.

With every round of the exercise pair, the training encompasses one lesser rep of each move; for instance, you move from a set of six to five…until zero.

You can also try density training where you pair opposing exercises for countdowns. For instance, kettlebell swing, pushups, and squat thrusts would work really well.

Do it!

Start by selecting your pair of exercises.

Perform six repetitions of the first exercise, then six reps of the other move. Go back to the first move and perform five reps then five more of the second exercise. Keep alternating until you reach zero.

In the subsequent workouts, add one rep to each exercise. If you want more countdowns, select a second pair from the list below, or just come up with your own pair of opposing moves.

Squat thrust, pushups

Kettlebell swing, squat thrust

Jumping jacks, pushups

Medicine ball side toss, medicine ball slam

As you get the hang of the above exercise, start the next:

Hurricane Workouts

This is essentially a workout protocol that entails lifting weights and interval training. We have three groups of exercises, called rounds in this type of workouts. Each round has an exercise that increases your heart rate, and a set of other exercises in between.

This design will allow you to keep your heart rate up throughout the workout (and burn significant amounts of calories) that typically lasts 16-22 minutes. Hurricane workouts have five levels and each one is an increased challenge. I have however prepared for you a sample routine you will work with below.

Note: This will require you to be more fit- if fit enough though, you can begin with this:

Warm up for the workout. For all rounds, do one set of each exercise and move on to the next exercise. Finish the whole round thrice before you move to the next round.

First round: Run on a treadmill at 10% incline, 10.5 mph for 25 seconds. Do a kettlebell Turkish getup about 4 times on each side of your body then 10 chin-ups.

Repeat this sequence thrice.

Second round: Run on a treadmill at a 10% incline, 11 mph for 25 seconds. Do 10 dips and a barbell rollout, 15 reps.

Repeat this process thrice.

Third round: Run on a treadmill at a 10% incline, 11.5 mph for 25 seconds. Perform the G,I row, 10 reps. Do the knee grab, 20 reps.

Repeat three times.

Negative Calorie Diet Tips

One thing you can be sure of is that the negative calorie diet will help you lose weight. The downside is that following a new diet can be challenging; hence, the below tips will make it easier:

Plan

Before you start any diet, you need to prepare. One good way to do so is by planning. This means getting your food ingredients and stocking up your fridge and pantry. As we have seen, there are varieties of foods you can eat. Thus, you may be at a loss as to what foods to buy more of if you don't have a plan. However, if you have a few recipes on hand, you can go ahead and buy the foods listed in the recipes. This will make your shopping easier. It will also ensure that you enjoy a variety of meals throughout the week.

Keep your goals in sight

One of the major blunders people make when they are on a diet is losing sight of their goals. Your goals are important. They are the reason you stick to your diet. Ask yourself why you're following the negative calorie diet. Write down the answers and place them in strategic locations. This way, you can remind yourself that you are on the right path and that you need to stick to it to enjoy the many benefits.

You can also motivate yourself by setting smaller goals and rewarding yourself whenever you achieve them. However, caution is needed. It would be counterproductive to reward yourself with high calorie foods. This will only set you back. But you can reward yourself with a new watch or with a pair of running shoes. This way, you will be happy to receive the rewards without compromising your diet.

Live your life

Your life should not be centered on your diet. Your diet should just be a small part of your life. It should not prevent you from enjoying other aspects of your life; you can still go out, socialize with others and exercise. In other words, you can and you should live your life to the fullest.

Yes, you may have to make a few changes. For example, you'll have to be careful to order negative calorie foods whenever you eat out. However, how is that different from ordering any other food? Live your life! The benefits that come with the negative calorie diet are just a bonus.

I need your help…

Thank you for downloading this book!

I hope this book was able to help you to know more about the Negative Calorie Diet and how you can burn fat and lose weight with this diet, the next step is to put what you have learned into practice and actually adopt the diet if you want to see those pounds coming off.

Finally, if you enjoyed this book, then I'd like to ask you for a favor, would you be kind enough to leave a review for this book on Amazon? It'd be greatly appreciated!

Clean Eating

Cookbook And Guide to Restore Your Body's Natural Balance and Eat Healthy

Introduction

I want to thank you and congratulate you for downloading this book,

Nothing in life comes close to the value of good health. Taking your health for granted will only lead to a life of compromise. You will not be able to enjoy life or be happy, as you will be pressured into thinking about your health.

Good health is a measure of how much you care about yourself. The more you care for yourself, the healthier you become and the happier you remain.

But this is often easier said than done. Most of us tend to lead busy lives that prevent us from focusing on our health. We tend to go through stressful situations that impact our bodies negatively. Add today's lifestyle encourages the consumption of junk and processed foods that can cause health to backtrack.

The need of the hour is to, therefore, pick up a diet that is wholesome and capable of enhancing good health.

When we hear the word "diet" we are often reminded of salads and soups that do not taste good. However, not all diets ask you to settle for bland food that is stripped of flavor. In fact, you do not have to follow a fad diet to enhance health, as a clean diet will do the trick for you.

A clean diet refers to subjecting the body to clean foods. Clean foods are all natural and those that are free from chemicals and toxins. Staving off consumption of such foods can put your health on the right track.

To give you a head start, this book has been written to teach you the meaning and importance of clean eating. It provides you with simple recipes that can be adapted to enhance good health.

The book has been designed to facilitate easy reading and you will find it simple to navigate through the different chapters.

Thanks again for downloading this book, I hope you enjoy it!

clarifying purposes only and are the owned by the owners themselves, not affiliated with this document.

Chapter 1: Importance of Healthy Eating

Health is wealth and it is extremely important for people to take good care of themselves. It is especially important in this day and age, when people tend to load their bodies up with junk and processed foods. Before we explain why it is important to eat clean, we will first look at its meaning.

What Is Clean Eating?

Clean eating refers to consuming foods that are natural and free from chemicals and preservatives. They include the likes of fresh fruits, vegetables, grains, legumes, pulses, oils etc. These are great for the body and will help you maintain good health.

Clean eating forbids the consumption of junk and processed foods. These are capable of negatively impacting your body. They promote the buildup of toxins that can, in turn, provoke illnesses. Clean eating subscribes to the principle that you should only consume those foods that are natural and which are good for the body.

Here are some of the rules that clean eating lays down.

- It is best to consume 6 smaller meals a day as compared to the regular 3 meals. Eating smaller meals can help the body to easily break down the foods and not feel burdened. But remember that it is the same 3 meals that will be split into 6 or 7 smaller meals, instead of 6 large meals.

- You meals should be made up of lean proteins and complex carbohydrates. Lean proteins help in the building of lean muscles. Lean muscles are tough to burn. You will be able to use up more energy while maintaining a lean body.

- You must incorporate a good dose of healthy fat in your diet. Not all fat is bad fat. Some fats help nourish the body and keep it strong. You must know how to incorporate the right fat in your diet.

- Clean eating stresses the consumption of 10 to 12 glasses of water per day. Water helps in flushing out all the toxins from the body. It also keeps you hydrated and enhances cell function.

- You have to eliminate all junk and processed foods from your diet. This includes the likes of take aways, restaurant foods, packaged foods etc.

- You must refrain from indulging in bad habits that can adversely affect your health. These include smoking, drinking etc.

- Although not a part of the diet, it will be best to avoid stress as much as possible. Stress can upset your body and negatively impact your health.

Benefits Of Clean Eating

Weight loss

One of the biggest complaints these days is being overweight. Every other person in the world complains about weight gain. But nobody really puts in the effort to shed their weight and people invariably end up making the same food mistakes as always. The best thing to do to fix this situation is adopt a clean diet. The diet will not only help reduce your current weight but also prevent any additional weight from piling back on. But you will have to follow the diet closely in order to experience positive results. The foods consumed as per the diet are capable of melting your current fat with the consumption of liquids draining it away.

Digestion

Digestion is one of the most important activities of the body. It is only through proper digestion that your body will be able to separate the nutritional elements from the food you consume and direct it to all the right organs. Although most of us think we have a healthy digestive tract, it is often not the case. It might look as though your digestive system is functioning optimally but there will be a few issues to tackle. Shifting to clean eating can help solve these issues to a large extent. The diet will promote liver and gut health, both of which are important to maintain a healthy digestive tract.

Illness

Many people fail to understand that illnesses tend to build up over time. The food choices you make, the levels of stress you experience etc. all have a bearing on your body's upkeep. If you stick to bad habits for too long then you are bound to suffer the consequences. The diseases might not show up immediately but will impact your health negatively in the long run. By switching over to clean eating, you will be able to stave off the majority of illnesses. These can include the likes of certain types of cancers, cardiovascular illnesses and brain disease. Clean eating also helps in controlling diabetes to a large extent. But you will have to carry on with the practice long enough to see these positive results.

Immunity

It is vital for your body to have proper immunity. Immunity helps in staving off the onset of illnesses. You will be able to lead a better life if you prepare your body to limit illnesses. Right from a common cold to digestive problems, it is vital to keep illness at bay if you are able to. Clean eating helps in this regard and keeps common problems from arising too often.

Brain health

Brain health is just as important as physical health. It is extremely important for people to stave off the onset of depression and anxiety. These mostly come about if an individual makes wrongful food choices and or leads a sedentary lifestyle. It will be important to address both in order to experience positive benefits. Consuming a clean diet helps in increasing the dopamine content in the brain. This helps in keeping stress and anxiety at bay. It also increases serotonin, which aids in keeping the mind alert and active. Brain health, in fact, can have a direct bearing on physical health. Your body will be able to burn away more fat if your mind focuses on this.

Hair and skin

The clean diet helps in enhancing both hair and skin health. The consumption of fresh fruits and proteins helps in strengthening the hair follicles and gives your hair a unique shine. Fresh vegetables and elements such as vitamin E aid in enhancing skin health. They increase the collagen content thereby making skin more elastic. You will feel youthful and develop a unique glow. You will also be able to fight away wrinkles to a greater extent. Consuming the right type of foods can reverse your skin's age and leave you feeling confident.

Nail and teeth health

The clean diet has a positive impact on nails and teeth. Shiny nails and bright teeth can make a person look attractive. One of the best ways to enhance this is by following a clean diet. The abundance of omega 3 fatty acids in the diet helps in strengthening nails and teeth. The diet also promotes the consumption of foods that are rich in vitamins C and E that aid in maintaining nail health. You will have less complaints as you age and be in a position to maintain good oral health.

Productivity

Adopting the clean diet can help you enhance productivity. You will be able to work better and get more out of your work life. The diet promotes the consumption of foods such as whole grains, fresh fruits and vegetables. These aim at increasing the level of dopamine in your brain, which is linked to productivity. They also decrease the cortisol level thereby enhancing brain function.

Better sleep

Sleep is one of the most important activities in life and yet many people fail to understand its importance. When you sleep, your body repairs itself from the inside. Defaulting on sleep will only lead to health issues. Many distractions tend to prevent people from falling asleep at night. The food they consume also has a big impact and can cause people to suffer from insomnia. Consuming clean foods can solve this problem to a large extent. The foods promoted through clean eating help in enhancing sleep and increasing the urge to sleep more.

Chapter 2: Foods To Keep Systems Clean

Clean eating involves the consumption of foods that are free from chemicals and additives. It focuses on ingredients that are natural and capable of enhancing the body's functioning.

Here are the clean foods to incorporate into your diet.

Foods To Include

Fresh fruits

Fresh fruits should be eaten on a daily basis. Fruits contain many types of vitamins and also antioxidants. These are required to keep your body healthy and prevent the onset of illnesses. They also help in keeping you looking youthful. You must aim at filling 20% of your plate with fruits. You can consume bananas, mangos, apples, grapes, pomegranates, watermelon, muskmelon, avocados, cherries, strawberries, lychee etc. Look for fruits that are in season and consume them as much as you can.

Fresh vegetables

You must consume fresh vegetables on a daily basis. One good way of incorporating vegetables is by picking 5 differently colored ones per meal. Say for example you pick carrots, peas, cabbage, tomatoes and yellow bell peppers. Try not to overcook them as they can lose their nutritional content. A simple salad or smoothie will make for a refreshing way to incorporate vegetables. You can consume tomatoes, okras, cabbage, cauliflower, beans, carrots, beetroots etc.

Lean proteins

Lean proteins are those that are free from fats and provide your body with the right amount of healthy proteins. They enhance your body's muscle building capacity. These muscles are tougher to burn and remain in your body for longer. There are many sources of lean proteins including fish, lean chicken and turkey, lentils, chickpeas, mushrooms, etc. You have to incorporate these into your diet as much as possible. It will be ideal to fill 30% of your plate with proteins.

Carbohydrates

Carbohydrates are an essential part of your diet. They provide you with adequate energy and assist with carrying out day-to-day activities. You must aim at consuming carbohydrates that are easy to break down. Brown rice makes for a better option as compared to white rice and whole wheat is good for your body as compared to white flour. A good trick is to have your heaviest meal just before working out so that you can successfully burn away the excess carbs.

Fats

It is a myth that fats are bad for your body. There are both good and bad fats and you must aim at increasing the good ones and decreasing the bad ones. The good ones are generally full of omega 3 fatty acids. These are important for brain and heart health. They contain a chemical known as DHA that is required by the body to remain healthy. A good source of omega 3 fatty acids is fresh water fish and flax seeds. Bad fats can build around your organs and turn into visceral fat. You have to avoid these in order to enhance good health.

Supplements

You can consider consuming natural supplements to enhance your health. Some of them include the likes of ashwagandha, Gingko Biloba and green tea. They will help in flushing out the toxins from your body while encouraging good health.

Food To Avoid

The clean eating diet asks for the elimination of certain types of foods that are bad for the body. Thoy aro as follows:

Junk foods

You have to avoid consuming junk foods as much as possible. These foods can cause your body to not function optimally. They include the likes of fast foods, fries, pizzas, burgers, deep fried foods etc. It might not be possible for you to completely eliminate them from your diet but you must aim at limiting them to just once or twice a month. You can also consider preparing healthier alternatives that will not be as imposing on your body.

Processed foods

You must also avoid processed foods. Processed foods are packaged foods that can contain preservatives and other chemicals. Right from chips to biscuits to cookies, to cakes and other such foods, you have to avoid them at all costs. Sodas are also prohibited as they can fill your body up with sugar.

Apart from these, you must try to avoid alcohol as much as possible. Smoking can also negatively impact you and you must kick the habit to cleanse out the toxins.

Chapter 3: Clean Eating Recipes

Breakfast Recipes

Veggie Deviled Eggs

Ingredients:

10 eggs

2 tablespoons cabbage, boiled

1 avocado

1 potato, boiled

5 tablespoons peas

2 teaspoons mustard paste

Salt to taste

Pepper to taste

Paprika to sprinkle

Method:

Add the eggs to boiling water and allow it to hard boil.

Meanwhile add the avocado to a bowl along with the potato, peas and cabbage and mix well.

Add the mustard, salt and pepper and mix until well combined.

Once the eggs are done, peel them and cut vertically.

Scoop out the yellow and add to the avocado mash.

Spoon the mix into the cavities and sprinkle the paprika on top.

Serve warm.

Healthy Muesli

Ingredients:

1 cup muesli of your choice

2 strawberries, chopped

1 banana, chopped

1 cup yogurt

2 tablespoons honey

1 tablespoon chia seeds

1 tablespoon sunflower seeds

Method:

Add the muesli to a bowl and add in the strawberries and banana.

Add the yogurt bowl along with the honey and mix well.

Add it to the muesli and mix well.

Add the toasted chia and sunflower seeds to it and mix well.

Chia Breakfast Pudding

Ingredients:

1-2 tablespoons honey

1/2 teaspoon vanilla extract

1/2 cup chia seeds

2 cups almond milk, unsweetened

Almonds for topping

Fruits like figs, blueberries, peaches and plums for topping

Method:

Mix the honey, vanilla, chia seeds and almond milk in a bowl, until well incorporated.

Allow the mixture to thicken in the fridge for a few hours or overnight.

Once frozen, stir well or add in some water in case you find the pudding too thick.

You can serve topped with fresh fruit and almonds.

Note: You can make your own almond milk by soaking almonds in water for 4 hours, then rinse and blend to obtain the milk. The pudding stores in the fridge for 5 days.

Main Meals

Chicken Wing Curry

Ingredients:

3 pounds chicken wings

1 large onion, chopped

1 jalapeno pepper, chopped

1 lemon, juiced and zested

2 cloves garlic, chopped

1 tablespoon coconut oil

1 cup chicken stock

Salt to taste

Pepper to taste

Cilantro to sprinkle

Method:

Add the onions to a pan along with the oil and sauté till brown.

Toss in the garlic and brown.

Add the peppers and sauté.

Tip in the chicken wings and brown it.

Add the lemon juice and mix.

Toss in the salt and pepper and mix.

Add the chicken stock and mix until well combined.

Sprinkle the cilantro leaves on top and serve.

Healthy Beef Stew

Ingredients:

1 large onion, chopped

2 teaspoons olive oil

1 large bell pepper, chopped

2 tablespoon jalapenos, chopped

4 garlic, chopped

2 teaspoons oregano

2 teaspoons coriander powder

2 teaspoons cumin powder

3 cups beef mince, cooked

4 cups spinach leaves

1 cup tomatoes, chopped

5 cups beef stock

1 lime, juiced and zested

Salt to taste

Pepper to taste

Parsley to sprinkle

Method:

Add the oil to a pan and toss in the onions and garlic.

Allow them to brown before adding in the bell peppers and sauté.

Add the oregano, coriander, and cumin and mix until combined.

Add the tomatoes, salt and pepper and mix well.

Add in the beef and beef stock and mix until well combined.

Cover and bring to a boil.

Once it does, add in the lemon juice and mix.

Toss in the spinach leaves and allow them to wilt.

Switch off the heat and sprinkle the parsley leaves.

Serve hot.

Easy Flat Bread

Ingredients:

1 cup wheat flour

Water to knead

Salt to taste

1 large carrot, grated

2 tablespoons vegetable oil

Method:

Add the flour to a bowl along with the salt and carrots and mix.

Add in a little water to make a firm dough.

Meanwhile, place a griddle on heat to warm up.

Allow the dough to rise for 5 minutes.

Make small balls out of it and roll it into circles.

Add a little oil to the pan and place one circle at a time to roast.

Flip once done.

Serve hot with your favorite stew.

Snacks And Desserts

Fish Sticks

Ingredients:

2 pounds cod or tilapia cut into strips

2 cups almond flour

4 large eggs

Salt to taste

Pepper to taste

5 tablespoons coconut oil

Method:

Add the flour and salt in a bowl and mix.

Add the eggs to a bowl and whisk.

Place a griddle on the stove to heat up.

Dip the fish in the eggs followed by the flour and place on the hot griddle.

Pour some oil on top and brush it over.

Flip the fish and repeat the same.

Fry on both sides until completely crispy.

You can add it to a preheated 350 oven for 10 minutes to further crisp it up.

Serve hot.

Peanut Butter Cookies

Ingredients:

2 eggs

2 cups peanut butter (preferably homemade)

2/3 cup brown sugar

1 teaspoon baking soda

½ cup unsweetened cocoa powder

1 teaspoon vanilla extract

2 cups peanut butter chips

Method:

Break the eggs into a bowl and whisk until light and fluffy.

Add in the peanut butter along with the sugar, soda, cocoa powder and vanilla and mix until well combined.

Add peanut butter chips and fold gently until smooth.

Grease a baking tray or add a paper to the bottom.

Add 1 tablespoon of the mixture on top and spread a little.

Place in a preheated 300 F oven for 15 minutes or until the cookies are done.

Allow it to cool down for 10 minutes and serve.

All Natural Flan

Ingredients:

3 cups coconut milk

5 large egg, beaten

2 teaspoons pure vanilla extract

2 tablespoons honey

2 tablespoons honey to caramelize

1 teaspoon lemon juice

1 tablespoon water

Method:

Add the coconut milk, eggs, honey and vanilla to a blender and mix until well combined.

Add the water, lemon juice and honey to a saucepan and allow it to caramelize.

Add it to a glass-baking dish and swirl around to coat the bottom.

Place this in a bigger tray with water in it.

Add the honey mixture to the dish.

Place in a preheated 350 F oven and bake for 15 minutes.

Allow it to cool down before serving.

Pecan Hotcakes With Berries

Ingredients:

1/4 teaspoon pure liquid stevia

1/2 teaspoon baking soda

1/2 teaspoon cinnamon, ground

2 teaspoons pure vanilla extract

4 whole eggs

8 ounce raw pecan pieces

Organic oil or grass-fed butter

Warmed frozen berries

Method:

1. Pulse the pecans in a food processor or blender to get a fine pecan meal.

2. Pour the pecan meal into a large mixing bowl and then whisk together stevia, baking soda, cinnamon, vanilla and eggs.

3. In a pan, warm some butter or oil and then ladle about 2 tablespoons of batter into the pan.

4. Cook the pancake until light and fluffy on both sides. Your hotcakes should fluff up when cooking.

5. In the microwave or pot, warm the frozen berries and then ladle them onto your hotcakes and serve.

Easy Salad Recipes

Traditional Egg Salad

Ingredients:

1/4 cup red onion, chopped finely

1/4 cup clean eating mayonnaise

8 eggs, hard boiled

Method:

1. Prepare the eggs by removing shells and then chop them into small pieces.

2. In a medium mixing bowl, put the chopped eggs, onion and mayo and combine well to blend. If necessary, add salt to taste.

Chicken Salad

Ingredients:

2 cups chicken, cooked and shred

1/4 cup walnuts, chopped

3 celery stalks, chopped

1 teaspoon rosemary

1 tablespoon vinegar

2 teaspoons olive oil

Salt to taste

Pepper to taste

Cilantro to sprinkle

Method:

Add the chicken to a bowl and toss in the walnuts.

Add the celery and rosemary and mix well.

Drizzle the vinegar, olive oil, salt and pepper and mix until well combined.

Serve with a sprinkling of fresh cilantro leaves on top.

Asian Vegetable Salad

Ingredients:

1/2 broccoli, chopped

1 large carrot, chopped

1 large cucumber, chopped

1 teaspoon sesame oil

1 teaspoon soya sauce

1 teaspoon White vinegar

1 tablespoon honey

1 tablespoon toasted sesame seeds

Parsley leaves to sprinkle

Method:

Add the broccoli, carrot, and cucumber to a bowl.

Add the sesame oil, soya sauce, vinegar, honey and salt to a bowl and mix until well combined.

Add it to the salad and toss until well combined.

Toss in the toasted sesame seeds and mix well.

Serve with a sprinkling of fresh parsley leaves on top.

Quinoa Salad

Ingredients:

2 cups quinoa, cooked

1 cup lima beans, cooked

½ cup mint leaves, chopped fresh cilantro, chopped

1 lemon, juiced and zested

1 tablespoon garlic powder

1 tablespoon honey

Salt to taste

Pepper to taste

Cilantro to sprinkle

Method:

Add the quinoa and beans to a bowl and mix.

Add in chopped mint leaves and lemon zest and mix until well combined.

Add the salt, pepper, lemon juice, garlic powder and honey to a bowl and mix well.

Pour it over the salad and mix until well combined.

Serve with a sprinkling of fresh cilantro leaves on top.

Chicken And Aocado Salad

Ingredients:

½ cup chicken, cooked and shred

1/4 cup carrots, chopped

1 large red onion, chopped

2 avocados, chopped

2 tablespoons balsamic vinegar

1 tablespoon olive oil

1 teaspoon mustard paste

1 teaspoon thyme leaves

Salt to taste

Pepper to taste

Parsley to sprinkle

Method:

Add the chicken to a bowl along with the carrots and onion and mix well.

Toss in the avocados and mix until well combined.

Add the vinegar and oil to a bowl along with the mustard, salt and pepper and mix until well combined.

Add this to the salad and mix well.

Sprinkle the thyme leaves and mix until well combined.

Serve with a sprinkling of fresh parsley leaves on top.

Egg And Tomato Salad

Ingredients:

2 eggs, boiled and chopped

1 zucchini, chopped

2 large tomatoes, chopped

1 onion, chopped

1 tablespoon vinegar

Salt to taste

Pepper to taste

Parsley to sprinkle

Method:

Cut the eggs into quarters and add to a bowl.

Add in the zucchini and tomatoes and mix well.

Toss in the onions and mix until well combined.

Add the vinegar, salt and pepper to a bowl and mix well.

Pour it over the salad and mix.

Serve with a sprinkling of fresh parsley leaves on top.

Spinach And Kale Salad

Ingredients:

1 cup spinach leaves, chopped

1 cup kale leaves, chopped

½ cup walnuts, chopped

1 avocado, chopped

Salt to taste

Pepper to taste

1 lemon, juiced and zested

Cilantro to sprinkle

Method:

Add the spinach and kale to hot water for 30 seconds.

Add to a bowl of cold water.

Remove and add to a bowl.

Toss in the walnuts and mix well.

Add the avocado and combine.

Add the lemon juice, salt and pepper and drizzle over the salad and mix.

Serve with a sprinkling of fresh cilantro leaves on top.

Fruit Salad

Ingredients:

1 red apple, chopped

1 green apple, chopped

1 orange, chopped

1/2 cup dried cranberries

1/2 cup chopped walnuts

1 cup plain yogurt

2 tablespoons honey

Method:

Add the apples and orange to a bowl and mix.

Toss in the cranberries and walnuts and mix.

Add the honey to the yogurt and mix until combined.

Pour it over the salad and mix well.

Serve cold.

Turkey Salad

Ingredients:

2 pounds turkey, cooked and shred

2 teaspoons garlic powder

2 teaspoons chili powder

2 teaspoons paprika

Salt to taste

Pepper to taste

1 avocado, chopped

½ cup corn

½ cup black beans

2 tablespoons salsa

1 tomato, chopped

1 onion, chopped

10 to 12 olives, chopped

Fresh cilantro to sprinkle

Method:

Add the turkey to a bowl along with the beans, corn and avocado and mix well.

Add the onion, tomato, corn and olives and mix well.

Add the garlic, paprika, chilli, salsa and salt to a bowl and mix well.

Pour this over the turkey and mix well.

Serve with a sprinkling of fresh cilantro leaves on top.

Couscous Salad

Ingredients:

1 large onion, chopped

1 cup spinach, chopped

1 cup garbanzo beans

1 cup olives, chopped

2 large tomatoes, chopped

2 avocados, chopped

1 tablespoon olive oil

2 cups couscous

1 tablespoon paprika

Salt to taste

3 cups water

Parsley to sprinkle

Method:

Add the couscous to a bowl along with the paprika, salt and water and allow it to swell up.

Add the onions, tomato, beans and olives to a bowl and mix well.

Toss in the avocados and mix well.

Once the couscous is done, add it to the salad and mix until well combined.

Serve with a sprinkling of fresh parsley leaves on top.

Smoked Turkey And Black Bean Salad

Ingredients:

2 cups cubed smoked turkey meat

4 cups field greens

1 teaspoon Dijon mustard

2 tablespoon cider vinegar

2 tablespoon olive oil

1 tablespoon minced garlic

¼ cup fresh cilantro: finely chopped

½ cup red onion, finely chopped

1 medium red bell pepper, chopped

1 cup shelled edamame, cooked and cooled

1 (14.9 oz.) can corn kernels, salt-free

1 (14.9 oz.) can black beans, rinsed and drained

Method:

Mix garlic, cilantro, onion, bell pepper, edamame, corn, beans and turkey in a bowl.

In a separate bowl, whisk together mustard, vinegar and the oil and then pour this mixture over the vegetables and turkey.

Toss to fully mix and then season using pepper and salt.

Once ready to serve, put equal amount of lettuce and then top with the vegetable and turkey mixture.

Beef Salad

Ingredients:

Sprinkle of oregano

1 chili, deseeded and sliced

2 handfuls lettuce

1 small cucumber, sliced

1 tablespoon crumbled feta

4 cups mushroom, sliced

2 cloves garlic, crushed

½ lemon, juiced

1 tablespoon olive oil

6 cherry tomatoes

300g Rump Steak, fully trimmed of fat

Method:

Drizzle the steak with a teaspoon of olive oil, small sprinkle of oregano and a clove of crushed garlic. Season with some salt and pepper too and set aside

Heat a griddle on high for about 5 minutes and then cook the steak on each side for about 3-4 minutes.

Put the salad ingredients in a bowl then sprinkle with sliced chili, squeeze of lemon, sprinkle of oregano, clove of crushed garlic and remaining olive oil. Use tongs to mix the ingredients thoroughly.

Remove the beef from heat and put it onto a plate. Allow it to rest while covered with foil, for 5 minutes.

Finally slice into strips before serving.

Artichoke And Asparagus Salad

Ingredients:

1 ounce shaved Parmesan cheese

1 pound medium asparagus, stems removed and cut into thirds

1 cup frozen green soybeans (edamame)

1 (14-ounce) can artichoke hearts, quartered

1/4 teaspoon pepper

1/4 teaspoon salt

1/2 teaspoon dried oregano

1 tablespoon lemon juice, fresh

2 tablespoons extra-virgin olive oil

1 garlic clove, peeled and halved lengthwise

Method:

Rub the insides of a salad bowl with garlic clove and then add in pepper, salt, oregano, lemon juice and oil. Whisk these until smooth.

Add in artichokes, toss the mixture slowly and allow to rest for some time.

Put the edamame into boiling salted water and cook for about 2 minutes.

Add in asparagus and cook the edamame and asparagus for 3 minutes. When crisp tender, rinse under cool water, drain and blot dry using a paper towel.

Add the edamame and asparagus mixture into the artichoke mixture, and then toss well to incorporate.

Finally distribute the salad among 4 individual plates. To serve, arrange shaved Parmesan over each salad.

Healthy Juices, Smoothies And Herbal Drinks

Spinach Juice

Ingredients:

2 celery stalks, chopped

½ cucumber, chopped

½ inch ginger, chopped

1 lemon, juiced

1 apple, chopped

2 cups spinach

Method:

Add the celery to a juicer and extract the juice.

Add cucumber and ginger and extract the juice.

Add the spinach, apple and lemon juice to a blender and whizz until smooth.

Combine it with the celery and cucumber juice and mix well.

Add in ice cubes and serve.

Cleansing Tonic

Ingredients:

1 teaspoon turmeric powder

2 carrots, chopped

1 apple, chopped

1 inch fresh ginger, chopped

1/4 cup orange juice

½ lemon, juiced

1 tablespoon honey

Method:

Add the carrots to a juicer and extract the juice.

Add the apple to the juicer and extract the juice.

Mix the two in a glass and add in the ginger.

Pour the orange juice and mix well.

Add in the lemon and honey and mix.

Serve cold.

Mixed Smoothie

Ingredients:

2 carrots, chopped

½ inch ginger, minced

1 green apple, chopped

2 stalks celery, chopped

½ cucumber, chopped

1 kiwi fruit, chopped

½ cup parsley, chopped

1 cup yogurt

1 tablespoon honey

Method:

Add the carrots to the blender along with the apple and ginger and whizz.

Add the celery and kiwi along with the cucumber and parsley and whizz.

Add the yogurt and honey and whizz until smooth.

Serve cold.

Beetroot Smoothie

Ingredients:

1 beetroot, chopped

2 carrots, chopped

3 stalks celery, chopped

½ lemon juice

½ inch ginger, chopped

1 cup yogurt

1 tablespoon honey

Method:

Add the carrots, beetroots, celery and ginger and lemon juice to a blender and whizz.

Add in the yogurt and honey and whizz until smooth.

Serve cold.

Orange And Strawberries Smoothie

Ingredients:

1 cup oranges, chopped

1 cup blueberries, chopped

1 cup orange juice

½ teaspoon salt

1 tablespoon honey

Mint leaves

Ice cubes

Method:

Add the oranges to a juicer and extract the juice.

Add the blueberries to the juicer and extract the juice.

Combine the two in a pitcher and well combine.

Add in the orange juice and mix until well combined.

Add the salt, honey and chopped mint leaves and use a muddler to crush the mint.

Add in ice cubes and stir.

Serve cold.

Digestive Drink

Ingredients:

1 cup Greek yogurt

1 cup buttermilk or regular yogurt

1 cardamom pod, seeds removed

1 small clove

½ teaspoon salt

1 tablespoon sugar

2 tablespoons mint leaves

2 tablespoons parsley leaves

Ice cubes

Method:

Add the yogurt and buttermilk to a blender along with the cardamom seeds, clove and blend until well combined.

Add in the salt and sugar and whizz until smooth.

Add in the mint leaves and ice cubes and whizz until smooth.

Serve with a sprinkling of parsley leaves on top.

Lemon And Mint Tea

Ingredients:

¼ cup lemon juice

1 cup mint leaves

1 teaspoon ginger, chopped

1 green tea bag

1 teaspoon black pepper

2 cups of water

1 tablespoon honey

Method:

Add the water to a pan and allow it to heat up.

Meanwhile, add the lemon juice, ginger, pepper and honey to a cup and mix well.

Add the tea bag to a cup and pour in the hot water.

Allow it to saturate.

Once done, add the tea to the juice and mix.

Serve hot.

Flower Tea

Ingredients:

½ cup rose petals, chopped

1 teaspoon black pepper

1 green tea bag

2 cups of water

1 tablespoon honey

Method:

Add the water to a pan and heat it up.

Add the petal and pepper to a glass along with the honey and mix.

Add the tea bag to a separate glass.

Pour one glass of water in the petals and another over the tea bag.

Allow them to steep for 10 minutes.

Mix the two together after straining the petals.

Serve hot.

Tomato Juice

Ingredients:

1 cup tomatoes, chopped

½ teaspoon ginger, chopped

½ teaspoon salt

1 tablespoon honey

1 cup mint leaves

Ice cubes

Method:

Add the tomatoes to the blender along with the ginger, salt, honey and mint leaves and whizz until smooth.

Add the ice cubes to a glass and pour the juice.

Serve cold.

Green Tea Spiced Tonic

Ingredients:

8 ounces purified water, near boiling

¼ teaspoon cinnamon

1/4 teaspoon turmeric

1 bag green tea

Method:

Into a tea cup, add in the teabag and the spices and then pour in the hot water.

Steep the tea and then remove the teabags. Stir to ensure that the spices are fully incorporated.

Super Juice

Ingredients:

Ice cubes

1 level teaspoon spirulina

1 ounce fresh wheatgrass powder or wheatgrass

½ avocados, ripe

½ cucumber, medium-sized

½ pineapple

2 apples

½ lime, peeled

Method:

Juice the apples, pineapple, lime and cucumber. Put the avocado in a blender and process until smooth then mix with the resultant juice.

Add the spirulina and wheatgrass and mix. Add in the ice cubes for a refreshing cold drink.

Purple Power Smoothie

Ingredients:

5 cashews

1 serving vanilla whey protein powder, unsweetened

1/4 cup pomegranate seeds

1/2 cup blueberries, fresh or frozen

1/2 cup raspberries, fresh or frozen

1/2 cup sweet cherries, pitted, fresh or frozen

1/2 cup water

Method:

Put the ingredients into a blender and process for around 60 seconds.

Serve and enjoy.

Kale Pear Smoothie

Ingredients:

5 raw cashews

1 serving vanilla whey protein, unsweetened

1 tablespoon lemon juice

1 cup pear

1 cup cucumber

1 cup kale

1 cup water

Directions

Place all the ingredients in a blender.

Blend until smooth then serve.

Clean Eating Tips

Clean eating is about making conscious food choices every day. You can do this by following the below tips:

Don't skip meals

Clean eating promotes a healthy lifestyle. This entails developing good eating habits. One habit you can form is eating breakfast. Breakfast gives you a boost in energy and allows you to start your day well. You should also make it a point to eat other meals throughout the day. This will keep you from raiding your pantry in search of junk food. If you want to eat some snacks, ensure they adhere to clean eating. There's no reason why you can't eat several meals and still enjoy a clean diet.

Cut down the costs

One thing many people complain about when they start clean eating is that, it is expensive. Well, it doesn't have to be. You can use many ways to cut down the costs such as:

- Use in-season produce

In-season produce tends to be cheaper than produce that has already gone out of season. This is because most retailers will be selling them. This brings costs down. If you make it a practice to eat such produce, you'll always have clean foods to eat without breaking the bank.

You can also buy fresh fruits and in bulk whenever they are in-season. This way, you can freeze them and use them later on when their production is scarce.

- Skip organic at times

You should definitely try to buy organic produce whenever you can. However, you should also know that there are times it is okay to skip organic. Foods such as avocado, cabbage, corn, pineapples and onions only absorb a small bit of crop chemicals. In this case, you can buy conventionally grown foods without feeling guilty about it.

- Shop in the frozen food section

You shouldn't neglect frozen food as you switch to clean eating. These fruits and vegetables are frozen straight from the farms and they retain their nutrients and antioxidants. In addition, many retailers have their own store brands of such foods and they often offer discounts. This means you can buy in bulk and save some cash.

The main idea is to go for foods that are good for you and still within your budget. You can also plan your meals to know what to buy. Meal planning allows you to greatly minimize wastage.

Drink water

You need to drink a lot of water throughout the day. Water not only keeps you hydrated but it also works to flash away toxins. This is good for your body and it meshes well with clean eating. Thus, you have to keep a bottle of water near you at all times and ensure you drink from it. Try to drink as much as 10 glasses of water each day.

I need your Help

Thank you again for downloading this book!

I hope you had a good time reading It. The main aim of this book was to educate you on the basics of clean eating and what it can do for you.

You need not follow a fad diet to remain fit. You have to change your lifestyle as a whole and make better food choices. I hope you take the advice mentioned in this book seriously and put in the effort to enhance your health.